Essential Oils for Wellness

Unlock Nature's Healing Secrets

Table of Contents

Chapter 1. Introduction

Discover a world brimming with aroma, wellness, and vitality with our Special Report on "Essential Oils for Wellness: Unlock Nature's Healing Secrets." Unveil an exciting journey into the universe of essential oils, rooted in age-old wisdom and complemented by contemporary scientific findings. This comprehensive guide will inspire you to transform your lifestyle with the therapeutic wonders of nature. From calming lavender to uplifting peppermint, every drop has a unique characteristic that can boost your mind, body, and spirit. Get ready to explore this riveting aromatic narrative that will make you want to dive right in. Illuminate your path to holistic wellbeing and make this valuable investment in yourself today!

Chapter 2. Exploring the Basics: What are Essential Oils?

Essential oils, often referred to as 'nature's pharmacy', are the potent, aromatic liquids extracted from various parts of plants.

Extracted primarily through steam distillation and cold pressing, these fragrant substances are more than just pleasant scents. They are deeply integrated with numerous facets of physical and emotional wellness, making them indispensable tools for holistic health.

2.1. Conception and Extraction

Whether it's the colorful petal of a blooming flower, the unripened peel of a citrus fruit, or the mysterious resin of a tree trunk, different parts of a plant conceal nature's precious biologically active compounds – essential oils. These oils have evolved in plants over millions of years as part of a sophisticated survival strategy. By attracting pollinators, repelling predators, and fighting off disease, plants use these chemical warriors – the essential oils – to thrive in a world of constant competition.

The extraction of these oils is an art and a science. Through two commonly used extraction methods, steam distillation and cold pressing, these concentrations are obtained, capturing the essence of the plant in its most prime state.

Steam distillation applies heat to the plant material, converting the essential oils into vapor before being cooled in a condensation chamber and then collected in a pure form. Meanwhile, cold pressing, more often used for citrus essential oils, mechanically squeezes the oil from the material with a precise combination of temperature control and pressure.

2.2. The Essence of Vitality and Therapeutic Benefits

With each oil encapsulating the aromatic profile, protective properties, and life force of the plant, essential oils become a direct link to the healing potency of the natural world. These volatile compounds interact beneficially with the body in numerous ways: penetrating the skin, engaging the olfactory system, and even having an internal effect when used appropriately.

Plants have served as humanity's oldest form of medicine, and their extracted essential oils are like concentrated healing allies. Each plant's key characteristics are reflected in its essential oil, from antioxidant to anti-inflammatory properties, from anxiolytic to antibacterial effects, and much more.

2.3. Essential Oils and Aromatherapy

Aromatherapy, a category of alternative or complementary medicine, uses essential oils as the main therapeutic agents to treat numerous health issues. Some of the most common uses of essential oils in aromatherapy include stress management, improving sleep, pain relief, mood enhancement, support for people who have chronic health conditions, and improving overall wellness.

Through methods such as inhalation, massage, or bathing, the essential oils reach our olfactory system or seep into our skin, assigning tasks to our body's cells with precision and impact. Interestingly, inhaling the aromatic compounds triggers our brain's limbic system, the part associated with emotion, memory, and state of mind, immediately impacting our emotional wellbeing.

When absorbed through the skin in dilution, these oils interact with the body's enzymes, hormones, and even immune system. It's like having an intimate and intricate conversation with nature herself through the language of biochemistry.

2.4. Quality Matters

To unlock the highest potential benefits, purchasing high-end, therapeutic-grade essential oils is crucial. Quality oils should be harvested from plants grown in their native or ideal environments, extracted without chemicals, and rigorously tested for purity and potency. Be aware that synthetic fragrance oils or adulterated oils lack the therapeutic benefits and may even be harmful.

2.5. Precautions and Safe Handling

Though essential oils carry immense benefits, improper practices or overuse can lead to adverse reactions. Dilute essential oils before topical application to avoid irritation, and consult with health practitioners, especially for internal use. Further, pregnant or nursing women, children, and individuals with existing health conditions should exercise additional caution.

2.6. A World of Splendid Diversity

The essential oil universe is astonishingly vast and diverse. From invigorating peppermint to calming lavender, from grounding sandalwood to uplifting citrus oils, each oil has an exclusive character. Understanding and appreciating each oil's properties, benefits, and applications can spark a fascinating journey toward phyto-aromatherapeutic space.

This journey into the basics of essential oils lays the foundation for your quest. As you explore further, you'll discover a world of nature's wisdom packed into tiny, fragrant drops, waiting to bestow you with health, vitality, and therapeutic bliss. Respect these potent extracts, use them with mindfulness and precision, to unlock an elevated way of living, and navigating the world around you.

Chapter 3. The Extraction Process: How Essential Oils are Obtained

The labyrinth of essential oil production begins in plant farms and ends in tiny amber bottles, with the delicate fragrance of nature captured within. This transformation involves a meticulous process, which demands care at every step. Understanding the extraction process broadens your view, helps you appreciate the precious oils more, and allows you to make safer and more effective choices.

3.1. Traditional Distillation

A time-tested and most widely used extraction method for essential oils is distillation. The procedure involves the use of steam to step-by-step rupture plant material cells to release the oils. These volatile oils get carried away by vapor and then cooled down in a separate chamber to form a mixture of oil and water.

The process begins with the collection of plant materials. Picked at the right time and carefully prepared, they are placed in the distillation chamber. Afterward, the chamber is sealed, and steam or water is introduced, either from the bottom or through a pipe running through the plant mass.

As the steam rises, it forces open the microscopic sacs containing the essential oil, and the volatile compounds are vaporized. The steam carrying the oil particles continues to rise into a cooling condenser, where it cools down to form a liquid. This liquid is a mix of essential oil and water, which is collected in a separate container.

Don't be misled by the presence of water. Because oil and water don't blend, the essential oil will float on the top, making it easy to separate using a separator.

Distillation methods can vary depending on the botanical material being used and the desired end product. Steam distillation, water distillation, and a combination of the two, 'hydro steam distillation,' are most commonly practiced.

3.2. Expression or Cold Pressing

Before distillation became commonplace, the cold-press extraction method was the favorite for obtaining essential oils from citrus fruits. Think oranges, lemons, grapefruits, and bergamot. Cold pressing is similar to the process used to extract olive oil.

The citrus peels are first carefully pricked to open the essential oil sacs. The fruit is then mechanically pressed to puncture the peel and release the essential oil. This oil is collected and centrifuged to separate it from the juice and other unwanted components.

Expression doesn't involve heat, meaning the natural characteristics of the oil remain intact, presenting you with an essential oil closest to its natural state, brimming with all of the fruit's vibrancy.

3.3. Solvent Extraction

Sometimes, heat and pressure are too harsh for the plant material, especially in the case of delicate flowers like jasmine or tuberose. For these sensitive botanicals, an alternative extraction method, solvent extraction, is employed.

In this process, a solvent such as hexane is used to dissolve the plant material and capture the essential oil, along with other soluble plant substances. The result is a thick mixture known as a concrete. When alcohol is added to the concrete, it dissolves out the essential oils to form an 'absolute.'

While absolutes are incredibly aromatic, they are not technically essential oils and can contain traces of solvents. As such, they are primarily used in perfumery, and care should be taken if using them for therapeutic purposes.

3.4. CO2 Extraction

The latest technology in the field of essential oil extraction is the method of CO2 extraction. In this process, carbon dioxide in its supercritical state (neither liquid nor gas) is used to extract the essential oils.

When pressurized CO2 is passed over the plant material, it acts as a solvent, breaking down the plant cells and carrying off the essential oils. The CO2 is then allowed to return to its gaseous state, leaving behind the oil.

Though CO2 extracted oils are expensive, they contain more plant compounds than essential oils obtained by other extraction methods, giving them more potent therapeutic benefits.

On this fascinating journey into the heart of essential oils, one common thread that stands out is the painstaking dedication and careful precision involved at each step of extraction. It's an intricate dance of art and science that harnesses nature's potent offerings to support your wellbeing journey.

From the distillation of potent peppermint or the cold pressing of zesty citrus fruits to the delicate solvent extraction of blooms like jasmine, each process is tailored to preserve the aromatic and therapeutic properties that these plants bring.

In the end, the understanding of the extraction process deepens your appreciation for each drop of essential oil. You become more intimately connected with the journey each bottle undertook, from rustic farms to your hands, becoming part of your journey towards wellbeing. Living with these potent oils can bring a profound connection to nature into your life that rejuvenates the mind, body, and spirit.

Chapter 4. Historical Background: The Use of Essential Oils Through the Ages

In the tapestry of human history, revered civilizations have time and again, embraced the inherent powers of essential oils. These elixirs condensed the vitality of plants into translucent droplets for various purposes; from spiritual enlightenment and medicinal applications to cosmetology.

4.1. The Dawn of Human Civilization and Essential Oils

During the early stages of human civilization, our ancestors formed their first bonds with nature. They discovered the rich scents of pines, the robust flavors in herbs, and the restorative qualities these contained. These primitive communities inadvertently kick-started the history of essential oils, although the process of distillation was yet undiscovered. They used plant parts directly, perhaps rubbing aromatic leaves on their bodies or using them in their food, thereby experiencing the benefits of these natural ingredients.

4.2. Ancient Egypt: Pioneers in Perfumery and Cosmetology

Centuries later, the ancient Egyptians played a key role in advancing the use of aromatic plant extracts. They created ointments and oils using innovative methods and employed these preparations in their elaborate rituals for the dead. They were also recognized for their use of fragrances in daily life, turning essential oils into the first perfumes. The scroll of Ebers, surviving from 1500 B.C, lists about 850 plant medicines, including oils from frankincense, galbanum, myrrh, cinnamon, and juniper.

Essential oils were also instrumental components in cosmetics. The famed Egyptian queens, Cleopatra and Nefertiti, reportedly incorporated essential oils such as rose, neroli, and frankincense into their beauty regimes.

4.3. Ancient India: Essential Oils in Ayurveda

Parallel to the developments in Egypt, the ancient Indian wisdom of Ayurveda (the science of life) was scripting its own aromatic narrative. Over 3000 years ago, this comprehensive healthcare system incorporated numerous essential oils for various therapeutic purposes.

A concrete testimony of this is the holy book of Hindus, the Rig Veda, which holds references to more than 700 aromatic plants and their medicinal applications. Oils like sandalwood and jasmine were recorded to have been frequently used not just for their therapeutic properties but also for spiritual enhancement during yoga and meditation.

4.4. Ancient China: The Birthplace of Traditional Herbalism

Circa 2800 B.C., the Yellow Emperor's Classic of Internal Medicine, the oldest Chinese book on healthcare, documented extensive usage of herbs and aromatic plants, indicating a likely use of essential oils. Notably, the Chinese were likely among the first to develop a method of extraction, although primitive, to obtain oils from plants.

4.5. Rome and Greece: Aromatherapy and Healing Practices

The Greeks took a leaf out of the Egyptians' book and developed their own aromatic practices. They praised the virtues of aromatic baths and massages with oil-infused ointments. The philosopher Hippocrates, also known as the 'father of medicine', documented the healing properties of approximately 300 plants, making a seminal contribution to the knowledge of herbal and, indirectly, aromatic medicine.

The Romans elevated the appreciation for aromatics to a new level. Their public baths used copious amounts of oils, not just for their scent but also for hygiene and therapeutic purposes.

4.6. The Middle Ages and Renaissance Period

The Middle Ages witnessed a brief decline in the use of essential oils due to oppressive religious sentiments, but it was also during this period that Avicenna, the Persian scientist, invented a coiled cooling pipe that made distillation of essential oils more efficient.

The Renaissance brought with it a renewed interest in botanicals and herbalism, spearheaded by figures like Paracelsus. Though contested, he was known to have used "essences" from plants, giving us the term 'essential oils.'

4.7. Modern Era: Scientific Exploration and Discovery

With advancements in science, the 18th and 19th centuries saw major strides in the extraction, identification, and usage of essential oils. Chemists began to identify key constituents and researchers studied their therapeutic properties more systematically.

The term 'aromatherapy' was coined by French chemist René-Maurice Gattefossé in the early 20th century when he discovered the healing properties of lavender oil on a burn.

Modern science continues to unravel the complex chemistry and the wide array of therapeutic benefits of essential oils, making them a subject of ongoing research.

Delving into the past helps us appreciate the journey of essential oils from primitive use to today's sophisticated applications. Just as our ancestors did thousands of years ago, we continue to seek solace and therapeutic benefits, bridging the gap with nature through these potent droplets. It is our testament to the ongoing relationship between mankind and the wondrous botanical world around us.

Chapter 5. Nature's Pharmacy: Therapeutic Properties of Essential Oils

Mother Nature's vast array of fragrant botanicals provides us with a treasure trove of essential oils, each with unique therapeutic properties. These tiny, potent droplets offer a host of physiological, psychological, and spiritual benefits, which we can harness for our health and wellbeing. This chapter delves deep into the therapeutic properties of essential oils, helping you understand their profound effects on our body, mind, and spirit.

5.1. The Fundamentals: What Are Essential Oils?

Essential oils are volatile compounds extracted from plants, including flowers, fruits, bark, stems, and leaves. Each oil holds the plant's fragrance, or "essence," thus earning its name. Beyond their diverse, pleasing aromas, these oils are well-regarded for their potential therapeutic benefits.

Let's explore how these botanical extracts can become an ally in our quest for improved health and wellness.

5.2. How Do Essential Oils Work?

These highly potent plant extracts interact with our bodies through direct absorption and inhalation. When applied topically, essential oils penetrate through the skin, making their way into the bloodstream. As for inhalation, the powerful molecules of the oils are inhaled into the respiratory system and then transported throughout the body.

It's essential to remember that the proper usage and dosage are crucial to ensuring the safe and efficient benefits of these oils.

5.3. The Therapeutic Benefits of Essential Oils

Each essential oil presents a distinct blend of therapeutic properties, determined by its unique chemical composition. For thousands of years, people have used these oils for their anti-inflammatory, antioxidant, antibacterial, antiviral, and antifungal properties.

Let's expound on a few well-loved oils and their therapeutic characteristics:

5.3.1. Lavender

Considered a pantry staple in the realm of aromatherapy, lavender oil is praised for its calming and relaxing properties. It's the go-to oil for dealing with stress and anxiety. Lavender essential oil can also alleviate sleep problems and improve skin health thanks to its potent anti-inflammatory and antiseptic properties.

5.3.2. Peppermint

Peppermint essential oil shines in its ability to re-energize and refresh. With its sharp, minty aroma, it can give a cognitive boost, improve focus, and support mental alertness. It's also commonly used to relieve headaches and soothe digestive issues.

5.3.3. Lemon

With its vibrant, uplifting aroma, lemon essential oil can stimulate the senses, invigorate the mind, and promote a positive mood. Its antiseptic and astringent properties make it valuable for skin care, while its detoxifying characteristics can purify the body.

5.3.4. Tea Tree

As a potent antimicrobial agent, tea tree essential oil is a popular choice for supporting immune health and combatting various skin conditions. Its antibacterial and antifungal properties are utilized for treating acne, dandruff, and fungal infections.

This merely scratches the surface of the multitude of essential oils gifted to us by Mother Nature. Each plant essence offers unique properties and meets specific wellness needs.

5.4. Blending for Maximum Benefit

Just as a symphony is more than the sum of its individual instruments, blending essential oils can create harmonious synergy that enhances their therapeutic value. Complementary oils can amplify each other's properties, resulting in greater health benefits.

Take lavender and peppermint, for example. When used together, they can provide soothing relief from headaches. Similarly, combining tea tree and lemon oil can create a potent blend for purifying and cleansing.

5.5. The Caveats: Essential Oils Safety and Precautions

Despite their natural origin, essential oils must be used with caution. Improper use can lead to adverse effects, such as skin irritation or allergic reactions.

Here are some safety guidelines:

1. Never apply undiluted essential oils onto the skin; always use a carrier oil for dilution.

2. Perform a skin patch test before using an oil you've never used before.

3. Keep oils out of reach of children and pets.

4. Avoid using essential oils if you're pregnant or nursing unless under the supervision of a health professional.

Essential oils offer a natural way to promote physical and emotional wellbeing. By understanding the diverse properties of essential oils, you can harness their therapeutic effects, enhancing your wellness journey with the fragrant gifts nature offers.

Remember, knowledge is power. The more informed you are, the better you can use these potent plant essences for your benefit. In the vibrant world of essential oils, there's always more to discover. So here's to your aromatic journey towards greater wellness and healing.

Chapter 6. Smelling Good: The Science of Aromatherapy

Aromatherapy, a centuries-old practice harnessing the power of plant extracts and essential oils, has been prized for its therapeutic properties throughout human history. Settled in the bosom of Mother Nature, this practice leans on the aroma of essential oils, the life essence of plants, known for their distinctive characteristics to uplift, calm, invigorate or balance the human mind, body, and spirit.

6.1. Understanding What Aromatherapy Is

Aromatherapy, also noted as essential oil therapy, employs natural oils extracted from flowers, leaves, bark, stems, and other plant parts to promote health and well-being. It has two primary mechanisms of action: the influence of aroma on the brain, particularly the limbic system through the olfactory system, and the direct pharmacological effects of the essential oils.

When the aromatic molecules reach the nasal olfactory epithelium, they get recognized and transduced into an electrical signal that journeys to the olfactory bulb and other brain structures, chiefly the limbic system. The latter is a group of brain structures responsible for our emotions, memory, and arousal, which elucidates why the smell is so potent in triggering memories and emotions.

On the other hand, the essential oils, being lipophilic, can easily permeate the skin and enter the systemic circulation, leading to potential therapeutic effects throughout the body.

6.2. The Making of Essential Oils

The process of extracting essential oils from plants is a delicate one. Most commonly, it involves steam distillation. The plant material gets exposed to high-temperature steam which vaporizes the volatile compounds (the essential oils). The steam carrying these vapors then cools down in a condensation system, turning back into liquid, from where the oils can be separated.

Some plants, like citrus fruits, undergo cold pressing or expression, methods chiefly used for peels rich in essential oils.

A less common but nevertheless important method is the use of chemical solvents, like hexane, that can pull out more delicate floral notes that might be destroyed during steam distillation.

6.3. Commonly Used Essential Oils And Their Properties

When delving into the realm of aromatherapy, you will find a vast variety of essential oils, each possessing unique properties. Here are a few gems from this treasure trove:

- Lavender: Known for its calming and relaxing properties, lavender helps in stress relief, sleep improvement and mitigation of migraines.
- Rosemary: Famously used for enhancing memory and concentration, and relieving stress.
- Chamomile: Cherished for its calming effects, chamomile is excellent for soothing anxiety and promoting sleep.
- Peppermint: An invigorating oil that can improve digestion, relieve headaches and boost energy.
- Eucalyptus: Effective in relieving sinus congestion and boosting

mental clarity.

- Lemon: Uplifting and detoxifying, lemon oil is great for mood elevation, and has antimicrobial properties.

6.4. Aromatherapy Applications

There are myriad ways to reap the benefits of essential oils. Inhalation and topical applications are the most commonly used methods.

During inhalation, volatile essential oil molecules get breathed into the lungs, providing both psychological and physical benefits, primarily through interaction with the nervous and endocrine systems. Diffusers are most popular for this purpose, circulating the aroma in your surroundings.

Topical application, on the other hand, lets the essential oils absorb through the skin, where they can interact with the body on a cellular level. Massaging with diluted essential oils or adding them to bathwater are examples of this method.

Safety is paramount when dealing with essential oils. They must normally be diluted with a carrier oil, like almond or jojoba oil, before skin application, as high concentrations can lead to skin irritations or allergic reactions.

6.5. Scientific Evidence Supporting the Use of Aromatherapy

Recent years have witnessed a surge in scientific studies aimed at validating the efficacy of aromatherapy and deciphering the mechanisms behind their therapeutic properties. Studies have shown potential benefits for various conditions, including anxiety, depression, pain, and several others.

Research on lavender oil, one of the most extensively studied, has suggested its effectiveness in sleep promotion and reduction of anxiety levels. In another study, rosemary oil was shown to enhance memory performance and increase alertness.

Studies on lemon essential oil suggest potential mood-enhancing attributes. Peppermint oil, too, has been seen in studies to reduce nausea and alleviate headache symptoms.

Though promising, more large-scale and well-controlled studies are needed in the area to establish concrete evidence.

6.6. In Closing: Essential Oils and Aromatherapy as Part Of Holistic Well-Being

Exploring aromatherapy is akin to embarking on a fascinating sensory journey where each oil contributes a unique tone to the symphony of wellness. Their scents can soothe, uplift, rejuvenate, or balance, and can offer a plethora of therapeutic benefits – shaping an integral part of a holistic lifestyle.

As science advances, so does our understanding of these plant extracts' power, taking us a step closer to harmonizing ourselves with nature. However, as we embrace their potential, let's not forget the importance of safety measures, proper usage, and individual suitability. May your journey with essential oils be enriching, serene, and saturated with wellness.

Chapter 7. Best Practices: Safe Use of Essential Oils

Diving into the fascinating realm of essential oils, it is paramount to understand the best practices for its safe utilization. The versatility and potency of these precious liquids necessitates careful handling and knowledgeable use.

7.1. Understanding Essential Oils

Essential oils offer a remarkable array of therapeutic properties, serving as important tools for promoting physical and psychological wellbeing. Derived from nature's bounty, these oils embody the unique chemical composition of the herb, flower, root, or resin from which they are extracted, thus encapsulating their healing qualities in a concentrated form.

However, to harness their therapeutic prowess effectively and safely, understanding essential oils, their nature, and their potential effects on individual health is crucial. While they can exert potent beneficial effects, their improper usage might pose significant health risks.

7.2. Essential oil Quality Matters

The suitability of an essential oil for therapeutic usage depends largely on its quality. It's therefore crucial to ensure your source of essential oils adheres to high-quality standards. Pure, unadulterated essential oils are potent and safe. They are often prepared through methods such as distillation, cold pressing, or resin tapping, with each oil bearing the distinctive chemical profile of the source species.

Look for oils that are 100% pure without additives or synthetic ingredients. Authenticity can sometimes be determined through the

Latin name of the plant species listed on the bottle, production method, country of origin, and whether the producer mentions "therapeutic grade" on the label.

7.3. Dilution is Essential

Due to their concentrated nature, most essential oils should be diluted before use to prevent skin irritation or other adverse effects. Carrier oils such as jojoba, almond, olive, or coconut oil are commonly used for dilution.

A typical guideline is a 2% dilution, which equates to about 12 drops of essential oil per ounce of carrier oil. However, this may vary based on age, health condition, and individual sensitivity. For instance, a 1% dilution (approximately 6 drops per ounce of carrier oil) is recommended for children, the elderly, and those with sensitive health conditions.

7.4. Safe Administration

There are three primary ways to use essential oils: aromatically (inhalation), topically (skin application), and internally (ingestion). Each method carries its own set of guidelines for safe use.

7.4.1. Aromatic Use

Inhaling essential oils stimulates the olfactory system, influencing the limbic system, which regulates emotions, heart rate, stress levels, and memory.

Utilizing a diffuser is the safest way to enjoy the aromatic benefits. Direct inhalation, which involves breathing in the oil directly from the bottle or a drop on your hands, can also be safe if done sparingly and with certain oils. Given their strength, direct inhalation may irritate the mucous membranes and should be avoided for certain oils like those high in phenols.

7.4.2. Topical Use

Essential oils can be applied to the skin for localized effects, but they should always be diluted with a carrier oil before application. Some oils, such as cinnamon or oregano, can cause skin irritation even after dilution, hence it is recommended to perform a patch test prior to full application.

Avoid applying essential oils to sensitive areas such as eyes, ears, or mucous membranes. It is also important to remember to wash your hands after application to avoid accidentally touching sensitive areas.

7.4.3. Internal Use

Although the internal use of essential oils is a controversial topic, some oils such as peppermint, lemon, and lavender are often used internally in a regulated manner. It is essential to adhere to dosage recommendations, and only ingest oils that are expressly listed as dietary supplements, with FDA-approved "Supplement Facts" labels.

7.5. Regarding Possible Allergies and Interactions

Essential oils can potentially cause allergic reactions in certain individuals, so it's advisable to carry out a patch test before regular use. This involves applying a diluted oil to a small patch of skin and monitoring for reactions.

Additionally, essential oils might interact with certain medications, so if you're on any kind of medication, please consult your healthcare provider before using them.

7.6. Pregnancy, Children, and Pets

Pregnant and nursing women should consult their healthcare provider before using essential oils. Similarly, they should be used cautiously with children, and some oils should be entirely avoided.

Pets, especially cats, can be highly sensitive towards essential oils. Never use essential oils on pets without the guidance of a veterinarian.

While essential oils offer a plethora of wellness benefits, they should be used responsibly. Knowledge, safety measures, recommended practices, and mindfulness in their usage are non-negotiable aspects of enjoying the bountiful gifts of these natural essences. By adhering to these guidelines, you'll be able to harness the robust therapeutic properties of essential oils safely and effectively.

The path to wellness is often a learning curve. However, determination and knowledge can enlighten us to make healthier, informed decisions, creating an optimum ambiance of well-being. The judicious use of essential oils can be one such journey, directed towards vitalizing our lives with the healing miracles of nature.

Chapter 8. Synergy in Action: Blending Essential Oils for Maximum Benefits

The captivating universe of essential oils extends far beyond their individual profiles. It introduces an innovative realm of formulation, blending—and yes, synergy. And therein lies the wonder: for when oils are meticulously paired, the outcomes surpass the benefits that the oils can offer singly. This harmonious combination, known as synergy, fosters magnified effectiveness.

In your journey towards embracing essential oils for wellness, understanding the concept of synergy is pivotal. It is through synergy that the true potency and magic of these oils unfurls.

8.1. Understanding Synergy in Essential Oils

Fundamentally, synergy denotes the mutual enhancement of each oil's potent constituents. It's an amplification of the therapeutic benefits, achieved through harmonized combination. The essence of the term synergy implies that the whole is unequivocally greater than the sum of its parts.

While isolating a single oil can offer a distinctive set of properties, creating a blend can formulate a grander, more comprehensive benefit. For instance, lavender oil has calming effects; eucalyptus oil plays a significant role in respiratory health. Combining these two can produce a powerful synergy that aids in calming respiratory irritation.

8.2. The Underlying Science of Synergy

Unveiling the scientific logic behind this phenomenon, synergy is predominantly based upon the interaction of different chemical constituents present in essential oils. Each oil has a unique chemical composition embodying various terpenes, esters, aldehydes, ketones, and more.

In a blend, when one constituent suppresses the adverse side effects of another or supports its medicinal activity, we observe a synergistic effect. For example, the monoterpene component of peppermint oil may enhance the absorption of the eucalyptol from eucalyptus oil, thereby intensifying the overall effect.

Furthermore, constituent groups within essential oils may also lead to synergy. A remarkable example is the interplay of linalool and linalyl acetate, both present in lavender oil. Independently, these compounds have relaxing properties; however, together they magnify this relaxation effect, demonstrating their synergy.

8.3. Crafting Synergistic Blends

The art of blending essential oils requires an understanding of oil categories and notes, as well as the oils' chemical constituents. It goes beyond picking oils with pleasing aromas; the oils' therapeutic profiles must be considered.

A good starting point is learning about oil categories. Essential oils are generally classified according to their herbal families such as citrus, floral, spicy, woody, etc. These groupings often interact well with each other and with oils within their own category.

Understanding notes is another key aspect. Every essential oil is labeled as a top, middle or base note based on its volatility or the rate at which it evaporates. Top notes are usually the first aroma you smell in a blend and evaporate quickly. Middle notes appear as the initial aroma starts to fade away, and base notes are typically the last to dissipate and provide depth and solidity to the blend.

Creating a balanced blend entails thoughtfully layering top, middle, and base notes. Ensuring each oil is represented ensures every layer of the aroma profile is experienced.

Next is contemplating the essential oils' chemical profile. Recognizing key constituents present can give clues to how oils may interact with each other. Linking oils that have common constituent groups can produce synergistic effects.

8.4. Synergy in Practice: Wellness-Oriented Blends

Energy Boost Blend

```
* 3 drops of Peppermint oil (Top note)
* 2 drops of Orange oil (Middle note)
* 2 drops of Rosemary oil (Base note)
```

Refreshing peppermint combines with uplifting orange and invigorating rosemary in this blend, perfect for invigorating mornings or combating afternoon fatigue.

Balance and Harmony Blend

```
* 3 drops of Lavender oil (Top note)
* 2 drops of Clary Sage oil (Middle note)
* 1 drop of Vetiver oil (Base note)
```

Known for their calming properties, lavender and clary sage mixed with grounding vetiver make an ideal blend for meditation or promoting restful sleep.

Through experiment and practice, you'll learn how these oils work synergistically and figure out your preferred blends. Every individual, just like every oil, is unique—let the principles guide you, but ultimately, let your instincts and preferences lead the way.

In conclusion, synergy in essential oils intensifies the oils' healing potential, providing opportunities for extraordinary wellness benefits. Understanding and harnessing synergy can empower you to create remarkable blends, amplifying the healing power of these wonderous botanical oils. Embrace the artistry of synergy and allow it to illuminate your path to holistic wellbeing.

Chapter 9. Taking the First Step: Incorporating Essential Oils into Your Daily Routine

The allure of essential oils lies not only in their enticing aromas but also in their multifaceted benefits that can significantly enhance your wellbeing. Embarking on this journey, you'll integrate small yet substantial changes into your daily routines, harnessing the power of nature to foster a healthier, more balanced lifestyle.

9.1. Understanding Essential Oils

Before we delve into how to incorporate essential oils into your lifestyle, it's essential to understand what they are and how they work. Essential oils are potent, volatile liquids derived from various parts of plants, including flowers, leaves, stems, and roots, through processes like distillation or cold pressing. Each oil encapsulates the natural aroma and healing properties of its source, providing a concentrated dose of nature's therapeutic benefits.

Viola et al. (2014) have highlighted essential oils' inherent characteristics, mounting clinical evidences for their chemopreventive activities, antimicrobial properties, and potential augmentation of drug therapy, confirming their multifaceted contribution to health and wellness[[Viola et al., 2014]].

9.2. Choosing Your Essential Oils

As a beginner, stepping into the realm of essential oils may seem daunting, given the myriad of options. Start by selecting a few oils known for their universal applications and versatility. Lavender for its calming effects, peppermint for invigoration, tea tree for its antimicrobial properties, and lemon for its uplifting aroma are a few good starters.

- Lavender: Deemed as the "Swiss Army knife" of essential oils, lavender is well recognized for its calming and soothing properties (Setzer, 2009). Use it to promote relaxation, alleviate anxiety, and enhance sleep quality.

- Peppermint: Its stimulating, invigorating aroma can uplift your mood, aid digestion, and enhance cognitive functioning (Tayarani-Najaran et al., 2014)[[Tayarani-Najaran et al., 2014]].

- Tea Tree: Known for its antimicrobial and anti-inflammatory properties, tea tree oil can serve as a potent home remedy for common skin conditions and minor wounds (Carson et al., 2006)[[Carson et al., 2006]].

- Lemon: Its bright, clean scent makes an excellent mood lifter and air purifier. Lemon essential oil possesses antioxidative properties and may enhance mental alertness (Kiecolt-Glaser et al., 2008)[[Kiecolt-Glaser et al., 2008]].

When selecting essential oils, consider their origin, purity, and how they're processed. Look for products that are 100% pure, meaning they contain only the desired aromatic plant compounds without added synthetic constituents.

9.3. Safe Usage and Precautions

While essential oils are natural, they're very potent and should be used responsibly. Improper use can cause irritation or adverse reactions. Always maintain a commitment to safety and heed the following precautions:

- Dilution: Pure essential oils should always be diluted before use. Carrier oils like jojoba, almond, or coconut oil are commonly used for this purpose.

- Patch Test: Before fully applying an oil, conduct a patch test on a small area of your skin to ensure there's no adverse reaction.

- Internal Use: Most essential oils should not be ingested. Seek out professional advice if you plan to use oils internally.

- Pregnancy and Children: Certain oils may not be suitable for pregnant women or young children. Always consult a healthcare professional before use.

9.4. Integrating Essential Oils into Your Daily Routine

Embracing essential oils doesn't have to be complicated. Here are simple ways to implement them into your daily routine, from morning till night.

- Morning Mood Booster: Start your day with an invigorating aromatherapy session. Diffuse peppermint or lemon essential oil to help kick-start your day with positivity.

- Skin Care: Add a drop of tea tree oil to your cleanser or moisturizer to promote clear skin. Lavender oil can help soothe irritated or sensitive skin.

- Work Focus: Counter afternoon fatigue with a peppermint oil inhalation. Its invigorating scent can help clear the mind and enhance focus.

- Relaxation and Sleep: In the evening, create a calming environment with lavender essential oil. Diffuse it in your bedroom to promote relaxation, or add a few drops to your bath for a spa-like experience.

9.5. Summary

Integrating essential oils into your daily routine carries the potential to profoundly impact your wellness journey. Remember, it's not a one-size-fits-all scenario. Experiment with different oils and modalities to discover what resonates most with your life rhythm. Begin with one step, and allow the organic growth of this natural lifestyle to enhance your mind, body, and spirit. Embarking on this healing journey with essential oils, you're strengthening your connection with nature, and in turn, with your most vibrant self.

With countless oils to explore, the journey can continuously evolve, mirroring your personal growth and opening doors to new possibilities for healing and wellness. As you step into this world of essential oils, you're not just taking a step towards a healthier lifestyle; you're taking a step towards a more balanced and harmonious you. Remember, each drop carries a unique, natural power, ready to support your wellness journey. Embrace this holistic approach, and let the transformative power of essential oils nourish your wellbeing.

Chapter 10. A Deeper Dive: Essential Oils for Common Health Conditions

The ancient tradition of using plants for medicinal purposes doesn't just pertain to botanicals ingested or used topically. A variety of oils extracted from these plants, often referred to as essential oils, encompass a myriad of health benefits and therapeutic properties. Let's delve into some common health challenges and how the healing power of nature be channeled through these oils to ease our ailments.

10.1. Understanding Essential Oils

Before we tread on the path to explore some specific oils, it's critical to clarify what essential oils are. Essential oils are concentrated plant extracts that capture the plant's scent or 'essence.' Obtained through distillation or cold pressing, the resulting aromatic compounds possess unique therapeutic properties.

With hundreds of essential oils to choose from, integrating them into your wellness routine might seem overwhelming. But when armed with a basic understanding and a touch of curiosity, unraveling their potential can be an empowering journey.

10.2. Lavender: The Tranquilizer

One of the most renowned essential oils worldwide, lavender, has long been adored for its calming and sleep-promoting attributes. Researchers suggest that the linalool — a terpene alcohol in lavender — can interact with the neurotransmitter system associated with anxiety, providing a calming effect. One can add a few lavender oil drops to a diffuser or pillow before sleep to promote healthy sleep patterns and reduce stress levels.

10.3. Peppermint: Breath of Fresh Energy

Peppermint oil can be a natural pick-me-up when you're feeling sluggish. The primary component, menthol, boosts energy, stimulates alertness, and improves concentration. It may also soothe digestive issues, working as an antispasmodic in irritable bowel syndrome (IBS) by relaxing the gastric muscles.

10.4. Eucalyptus: Nature's Decongestant

Best known for its role in respiratory health, eucalyptus oil has proven to be a potent decongestant, relieving symptoms of common colds, coughs, and sinusitis. The eucalyptol in this oil can break up mucus making it easier to expel, doing wonders for nasal congestion.

10.5. Tea Tree: Skin's Best Friend

Tea tree oil, or Melaleuca, is widely known for its antimicrobial, antiseptic, and anti-inflammatory properties. It can be used topically to treat a variety of skin conditions, including acne, psoriasis, and dermatitis. Studies suggest it's as effective as benzoyl peroxide in treating acne, without the associated side effects.

10.6. Rosemary: The Cognitive Enhancer

Researchers associate rosemary oil with an improved cognitive function. It may improve concentration, memory, and mental alertness. Furthermore, its camphor content assists in relieving muscle pain and spasms making it a useful addition to massage oils.

10.7. Chamomile: The Peace Promoter

Chamomile essential oil, particularly Roman chamomile, is best for stress, anxiety relief, and promoting peaceful sleep. Researchers link its chief compound, chamazulene, to anti-inflammatory and soothing properties, substantiating its use in soothing skin irritations.

10.8. Important Safety Considerations

Essential oils can have amazing benefits when used properly, but they are potent substances that require caution. Always conduct a skin patch test before applying oils topically to check for potential allergic reactions. Also, remember that essential oils should generally be diluted in a carrier oil or diffused before use. Pregnant women, individuals with specific health conditions, and children should always consult healthcare professionals before introducing essential oils into their routines. In addition, internal use of essential oils should be guided by a professional only, as it may have potential risks.

10.9. Incorporating Essential Oils into Daily Life

In your journey of integrating essential oils into your daily regimen, consider two main factors: the particular health condition you aim to address, and the method of application. Methods could include diffusing, applying topically, or adding to baths, beauty products, or cleaning supplies.

An exploration of essential oils is really an exploration of nature and its monumental benefits. By integrating these health-supporting, aromatic wonders into your lifestyle, you can foster a more mindful and wellness-centered existence. Remember, while essential oils can offer great support and relief for various common health issues, they are not meant to replace appropriate medical treatment.

Chapter 11. Future Outlook: The Role of Essential Oils in Modern Health and Wellness

The integration of essential oils into modern health and wellness practices is not only a trend but also a testament to the merits and potentials these natural substances possess. It echoes the increasing public sentiment towards more natural, less invasive, and more holistic approaches to wellbeing.

11.1. The Intersection of Traditional and Contemporary Medicine

Historically, mankind has harnessed the healing properties of essential oils derived from a variety of plants. Traditional medicine systems worldwide, from Ayurveda in the east to Herbalism in the west, have employed these oils to treat various maladies. Fast forward to today's age, where scientific exploration is collating empirical evidence to support these anecdotal claims, transforming essential oils from mere alternatives into credible health solutions.

The advent of aromatherapy, a practice that uses aromatic essential oils medicinally to improve physical and psychological wellbeing, has underscored the role of these oils in modern health care. A fascinating mix of empirical science and traditional wisdom, aromatherapy advocates for the use of oils such as lavender for relaxation, peppermint for increased alertness, and eucalyptus for respiratory health, among others. These pioneering applications of essential oils have laid a precedent for their role in modern health and wellness, a trajectory only set to surge upwards.

11.2. The Growing Pharmaceutical Interest in Essential Oils

No small part of the future pertains to pharmaceutical industries recognizing the potential benefits of essential oils in developing new treatments. Numerous studies show promise in essential oils' antimicrobial, antifungal, antiviral, and anti-inflammatory properties, making them suitable for inclusion in topical treatments and medications.

One such example is tea tree oil, prized globally for its potent antiseptic properties and its ability to treat wounds. Then there's oregano oil, with its powerful antiviral properties, and peppermint oil, used extensively in addressing gastrointestinal discomfort. Modern research shows these oils can be used effectively in treating conditions traditionally handled by over-the-counter medicines or prescriptions.

Pharmaceutical reconciliation of these natural substances offers enormous potential for drug patenting, creating enormous industrial interest. This commercial potential, in turn, feeds into expanded research into these oils and their therapeutic benefits.

11.3. Essential Oils and Preventive Medicine

Preventive medicine focuses on the health of individuals, communities, and defined populations. Its aim is to protect, promote, and maintain health by preventing disease, disability, and death. Essential oils, with their broad range of beneficial properties, find a natural place within this framework, contributing to health preservation.

For instance, oils boasting anti-inflammatory qualities such as frankincense, and oils with restorative properties such as sandalwood, are demonstrated to help maintain or restore health. On a socio-cultural level, the use of these oils aligns with a trending shift towards natural, preventive-based health habits.

11.4. Essential Oils and Mental Health

The link between essential oils and mental health is a topic of growing interest within the scientific, health, and wellness communities. The potential for essential oils to impact mental health, particularly concerning stress, anxiety, and depression, is being examined seriously by modern researchers.

In aromatherapy, oils like lavender, chamomile, and jasmine are often recommended to ease stress and anxiety, promoting a sense of calm. As the prevalence of mental health disorders globally continues to increase, the need for diverse, accessible, and natural treatment options soars. Thus, a broader acceptance and implementation of essential oils appear increasingly likely.

The future of essential oils in modern health and wellness seems bright. With burgeoning research corroborating traditional knowledge and practices, the integration of essential oils into modern preventive and therapeutic medicine is not far off.

While conventional medicine will continue to be necessary, the complementary role of essential oils provides a wider array of options, emphasizing the significance of personalized care—and subsequently, a more holistic outlook on health and wellness. Make no mistake, as we sail forth into the future, essentials oils will become increasingly embedded in our wellness regimen, paving the way for a harmonized, more natural path to wellbeing.

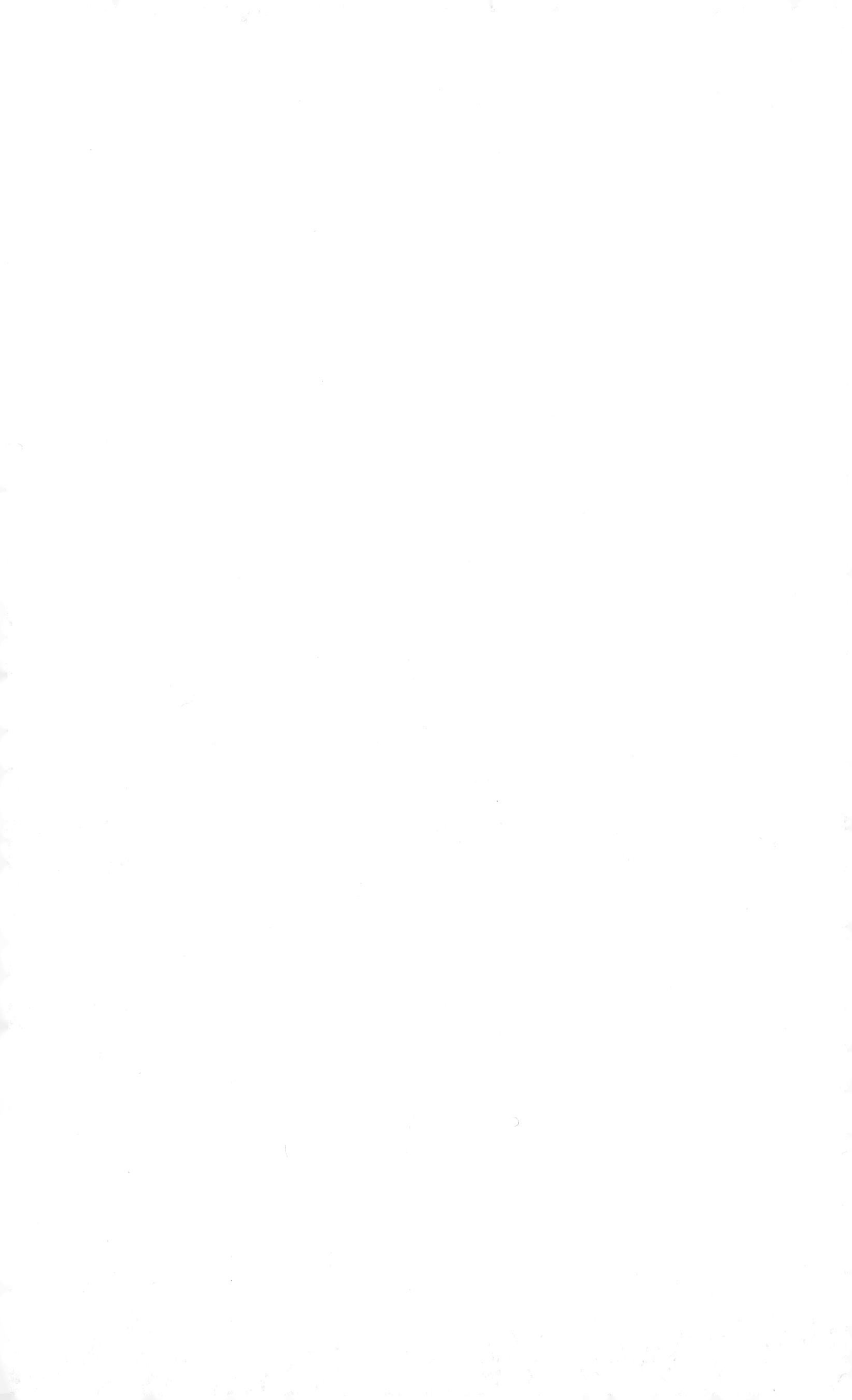